WEIGHT LOSS THE PERFECT KETO DIET COOKBOOK A SOURCE OF QUICK-ACTING NATURAL RECIPES FOR LOSS OF MORE THAN 9KG PER WEEK.

By

Ronnie Rey

Table of Contents

Introduction

This book includes the best natural delicious recipes you can now relax and enjoy all the benefits of a stress-free diet.

Chapter 1

The key to success in choosing a new diet is easy and how to maintain it for a whole month.

Chapter 2

Some general tips and guidelines to follow during the period of slimming.

Chapter 3

The nutritional basis for preparing my food systems is suitable for your skill in cooking.

Chapter 4

Some vegetables, fruits foods and drinks should, be eaten within a full week to get good results.

Chapter 5

A detailed feed system consists of breakfast, lunch and dinner for a full seven days.

Chapter 6
More than 30 natural healthy recipes for quick weight loss.

Chapter 7
Supplementary advice on diet, sleep and its relationship to low weight.

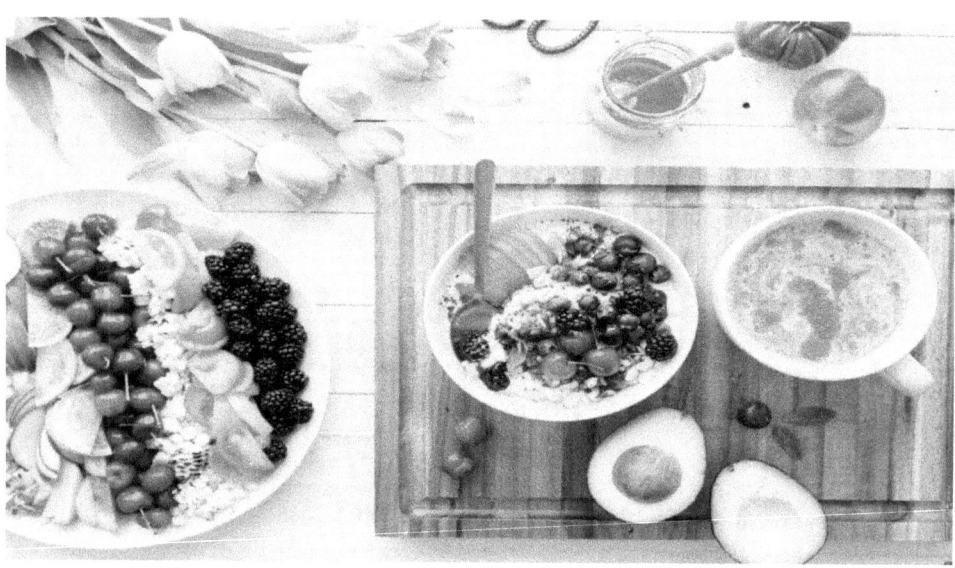

Hello, everybody before we start I have some question for you ?
- Are you overweight ?
- Are you searching for healthy life ?
- Can t wear your favorite clothes ?
- Always feel tired or out of energy ?
- Have some health problems due to over weight ?
- Tried many regimens with no result ?

If you answer is YES for one or more questions se you are in the right place and right time to change that forever.

Beginning another eating regimen might be troublesome in the event that you don't have a decent arrangement for what you can eat. This is the book you are searching for, I have done all the cooking and arranging estimations for you, I picked you simple to utilize suppers to make your taste heavenly.

Chapter 1

The key to success in choosing a new easy diet is how to maintain it for a whole week.

This book incorporates all formulas with various sugars and proteins. You would now be able to unwind and appreciate every one of the advantages of a tranquil eating regimen however the way to progress lies in deciding and looking after parity.

1-Balancing Your Plate, A reasonable plate is vital in any eating routine to guarantee you get enough supplements went for getting a sound segment of fat protein and starches in every feast.
2-Build Your Basis An eating regimen dependent on a wide scope of vegetables and entire vegetables. This should shape the premise of your dinner and spread 70% of your dish. From here you can include solid fats and pick a protein.
3-Skip the desserts – The eating regimen expels a ton of refined sugars and prepared sustenance's. With an emphasis on entire common nourishments, change the cakes with an organic product with a little yogurt.
4-Keep sound fats - not at all like fats that make you fat. Sound fats would already be able to give a wide scope of medical advantages and add to weight reduction. Among the fundamental components in the eating regimen is the utilization of great olive oil, which can be counteracted for coronary illness and give hostile to maturing properties.

5-Reduce meat utilization - The eating regimen centers vigorously around plant proteins and fish. Albeit moderate bits of creature protein are incorporated. Red meat ought to be kept at any rate and poultry ought to be eaten respectably.

Beginning another eating regimen does not need to debilitate and speaks to an extraordinary open door for innovativeness in the kitchen. Utilizing these critical tips ought to be a decent beginning stage for structure of your new eating routine.

Chapter 2

Some general tips and guidelines should be followed during the slimming period.

I need to impart to you the key to getting a thin body without infection is to walk 40 minutes consistently and this is the exhortation of global specialists.

On the off chance that you have just taken a gander at the fridge, seeking after motivation, let my book help you dispose of this inclination, on the grounds that every container contains numerous flavorful conceivable outcomes, additionally put the substance of the cooler by disclosing how to turn your most loved fixings in these delightful and tasty formulas.

A speedy acting eating regimen loses 9kg for each week here are some broad tips and rules to pursue when eating a quick processing eating regimen.

-Drink no less than 6 glasses of water multi day.

-Anise and hibiscus can be taken with the expansion of sugar substitutes.

-Tea and espresso can be taken without sugar.

-It is taboo to drink a wide range of carbonated water

-It is illegal to eat baked goods.

In the event that you feel hungry, you can eat any measure of cucumber or lettuce each one in turn.

Chapter 3

The nutritional basis for preparing my food systems is suitable for your cooking skills.

It merits referencing that numerous natives wish to know the privileged insights of the wholesome bases to be mulled over in the readiness and plan of nourishment regimens since they are viewed as the most vital purposes behind satisfaction and achievement and mental dependability, the young lady toward the start of her childhood need to look alluring and rich polish, and develop ladies need to seem granular appearance Her significant other, her kids, her companions, her relatives, her associates and partners at work, lodging and at the club, just as representatives whose appearance is a piece of their prosperity. Extreme Rsm to show up as tolerable before their customers, and the old to give fitting surfaces to them and spare them from corpulence or meager - to keep up their wellbeing and imperativeness.

It ought not to be overlooked that the sensational upset in correspondence right now has essentially decreased endeavors to do anything contrasted with what has officially gone on. Moreover, the phenomenal multiplication and expanding interest for inexpensive food abstains from food that contain the high cost thickness that has caused In the enduring of numerous natives and youngsters specifically, kids and grown-ups from stoutness and its chaperons from basic wholesome infections, for example, diabetes, hypertension, unpleasant joints, atherosclerosis, expanded cholesterol and disappointment As well as the event of a feeling of supported pressure, poor ovulation and the rate of gallstones and the rate of strikes in the menstrual cycle.

In light of the above mentioned, we should think about the nourishing reason for the planning of sustenance regimens, of which we will make reference to the most essential ones, for instance, however not constrained to the accompanying:

1 - We recommend that when you feel hungry drinking water and this has a great effect on eating; this feeling may be due to thirst and not hunger.
When applying all types of meals, it is recommended to take 6 glasses of water a day, two cups of water when waking up in the morning, two cups of water between breakfast and lunch, and drink two cups of water between lunch and dinner.
Drink as much water as possible. Research has shown that drinking two cups of water in the morning.
May help every woman to raise the level of low blood pressure, despite the importance of drinking water, especially in the warm climate, but excessive eating has serious consequences, especially if continued for a long period of time because it may lead to Control of water poisoning, which disrupts biological processes related to water in the body.
Therefore, athletes are not advised to take large amounts of water and fluids before feeding them a thirst for fear of drought caused by the loss of a large number of body fluids because of drinking plenty of water during running or other sports reasons, including sweating. The sudden death of some athletes due to hypothyroidism in the blood.

2 - Recommend reducing the use of the salt table because it works to store water in the body.

3 - The need to exercise at least daily so as not to lose muscle fitness If you follow a diet helps you to lose weight quickly, there may actually occur many when you stop following this diet, your body gets fat and loses muscle as well.

4 - The combination of the best components of diets that rely on reducing carbohydrate and fat may be more effective for long-term weight loss.

5 - Note that girls and women follow a strict diet such as the chemical diet triangles melon and banana leads to anorexia and this means that many teenage girls and some women around the world to refrain from obesity or overweight, which can lead to a defect in the body organs Because of the severe shortage of many nutrients that may stretch, this imbalance sometimes occurs after marriage or the desire to have children and perhaps for their children later, if a healthy and balanced diet is not applied, we recommend these teenage girls, ladies and all people To realize that the best diet system is to eat all foods, but in moderate amounts without wasteful with a lot of eating fresh and cooked fruits and vegetables and reduce and not refrain from eating sugars, sweets, oils and fats with the exercise of walking.

6 - A diet with high amounts of protein is often more effective to lose weight .
From a diet based on low-fat foods alone because the protein-rich foods make the person feel full and absorb the body from the energy resulting from the heat and it leads to the loss of less muscle while not accumulate new layers of fat quickly as soon as Stop following this diet.

7 - Low-carbohydrate diets, which are widely excluded from eating fruits, vegetables and grains, initially reduce weight better than low-fat diets, but in the long run are not better and may have side effects Diarrhea, muscle weakness, and dehydration.

8 - Carrot and radish syrup helps treat liver strikes and eliminate plaque
Fatty and kidney stones in the body and reduce the proportion of cholesterol.

9 - Eat a large dish of green salad full of different types of vegetables colored before Start eating the main dishes for about 20 minutes helps reduce the number of calories contained in the body with each meal, preferably include some lettuce and carrots section Tomatoes, cucumbers, celery, parsley and dill with a small amount of low-fat sauce.

10 - Pineapple is one of the best fruits that reduce weight especially as it helps digestion Proteins and fat burning.

11 - Walnuts although it is high in fat but contains the substance of serotonin, which helps to feel full quickly, as well as it causes moderate mood.

12 - Take 50 grams of dried grape leaves after immersion in cold water and lemon and leave on low heat until boiling and then filtered and eating three cups of it after food reduces weight.

13 - The belief that drinking hot water in a diet helps to burn fat is unfounded, preferably drinking water at a mild temperature is not hot, and it is recommended to distribute water rations throughout the day in the diet. Drink two cups of water after waking up before breakfast before dinner for a quarter of an hour, after eating for half an hour, do not drink water during meals so as not to relax gastric juice, leading to delayed food in the stomach, leading to indigestion, the body extracts acetone And ketones, which are toxic substances that cause depression, lethargy, laziness, depression, nervousness and lack of sleep during dieting.

14 - Note that in solid systems lose 5 kg of body weight in the first week following, half of this amount of water because 70% of the fat cells consist of water so what happens during these systems is low blood glucose, fat cells and sodium potassium levels in Body, the body withdraws large amounts of water, leading to dry skin, the appearance of wrinkles, low blood circulation and lack of pressure to avoid it, appropriate amounts of water, also affects the kidney function during the adoption of solid meals less than 3 liters of water a day.

15 - Raisins in milk to take advantage of insulin in raisins increase the absorption of calcium milk and maintain the health and safety of colon and bone by increasing the amount of insulin to absorb calcium by 20%.

16 - In the case of diets that help to gain weight in thinness, you should take four tablespoons of black honey a day because black honey and medicines are rich in calories and also contain simple materials easy to digest and absorption, in addition to being useful in terms of treatment as a bacteria against the incidence of poverty Blood and constipation, helps digestion and effective antioxidants, calms nerves and prevents premature aging.

17 - advised when using a diet using vinegar, apple cider vinegar, it reduces the proportion of fat in the body, which helps to treat the body more efficiently by converting complex fats to simple fats, easy to disassemble and digestion and leads to the elimination of feeling numbness.
This diet is based on the use of apple vinegar to reduce weight by dissolving a spoon of medium in a cup of warm water and drink after the meal is not recommended to eat excessive apple vinegar because it can lead to many health problems such as stomach infections and liver and change the acidity of blood, and recommended to add a small amount of Vinegar on the green salad dish to reduce body fat without harm to health, and is always advised to add vinegar in small quantities within meals and not on empty stomach.

18 – It is the miracle of dietary carnitine compound to achieve fitness and get rid of obesity where the fat is taken from inside the body and put into combustion by the furnace in each cell of the human body, which in turn is burned and converted to energy instead of aggregation, which helps to resist obesity and give vitality Fortunately, these common meals are available in our daily lives, such as those that include legumes and grains together in a single meal such as kosher or rice with lentils, as well as sesame seeds, with peanuts, white pulp, oranges, and bananas, to get the body burning calories Exclusive.

19 – For a successful diet, it is best to get rid of a certain number of kilograms in the first stage of the diet. When you do this, you can complete the disposal of the remaining kilograms in stages. Keep in mind that slow chewing food is important to the success of any diet because eating quickly and without chewing does not make you feel full quickly and cause gastric clots that cause obesity.

As well as the need to eat meals at specific times of the day because it helps regulate the secretion of hormones that cause hunger, and advised to eat five small meals of food during the day so as not to feel hungry, especially in the evening.

It is recommended to eat 3 dishes because it helps to feel that the fibers in it is not recommended to avoid certain types of food such as pasta or bread because the body needs but must be less than the fat used in the preparation and caution in the weight of meals in general with eating fish twice a week, As well as brisk walking for 40 minutes a day.

20 - A diet of one type is one of the biggest risks of dieting, which does not scientifically depend on food balance, because it severely weakens women's immunity and makes them vulnerable to disease. The immune system is one of the most important devices that protect the body from dangers, whether outside the body such as microbial infection or inside the body is like tumors. As a result, eating high-protein balanced lunch, eating fresh vegetables and fruits to contain vitamins, especially antioxidants that kill dead particles that cause premature aging, tumors, and atherosclerosis, is important when dieting is low.

21 - Eating white bread and pastries is a list of foods that cause obesity .
It was found that people who eat larger amounts of white bread are ranchers and obesity rates higher than those who eat the pills because the egg white turns into sugar once it enters the body, which makes insulin levels rise in
The body to burn the amount of sugar in the blood and stored in the cells of the body which is above the stomach and is the perfect place to burn these amounts of excess sugar. Therefore Eating brown bread is better when following food regimens because it avoids humans the phenomenon of the rumen as well as it protects the body from heart disease and diabetes.

22 - It was found that the consumption of large amounts of energy foods such as whole grains and fruits Vegetables do not increase the calories within the body because it is whenever The consumption of these foods much as a person felt fullness and fullness, but increase the total number of calories consumed, as well as it reduces the desire of the human to eat fatty foods or entertainment or even excessive eating.

23 - Note that a moderate diet helps the body to get rid of excess weight, and steadfastness for many years keeps his health and safety. It seems that the diet of yoyo reduces and weakens the immune system of the body. Because women who follow the diet at intervals are suffering from the ease of taking their bodies to viruses and microbes, and thus easily susceptible to many diseases because this oscillation weakens the immune system of the body.

The yoyo is a term used by dietitians for women who have been on a diet for weight loss.

When this is achieved, they return to their normal diet and the body regains the weight it lost with several extra kilos.
This yo-yo system is repeated before occasions requiring clothing that needs to get rid of excess weight. Perhaps the best diet recommended is the one that depends on a small amount of sugar and fat, and a large number of vegetables and fruits, in addition, to follow and exercise some simple exercise because follow such The system as a way of life ensures that women are healthy and achieve the required agility at the same time.

24 - Take extreme care to follow the harsh diet of obese people of the excess
Weight because it brings serious health damage as it exposes them to depression As a result of the deprivation of many types of food in addition to exposure to low blood pressure and because of the acute lack of protein because of this diet.

25 - It should not be forgotten that the popular foods of the Muslim peoples in general and of Egypt, in particular, have great health benefits such as condensed beans, lentils and peanuts because they contain substances rich in arginine that reduce cholesterol and also help to protect blood vessels, Arginine is also found in dairy products. Therefore, these foods should be included in weight-reducing diets.

This is to eat dairy products full fat and rich Calcium and linoleic duplications work to rid the body of fat and reduce weight Overload are unlike what is common among people.

Therefore buffalo milk is characterized by it high fat compared to low - fat bovine gravy is classified among the most useful foods in Treatment of obesity despite its high content of fat, but that fat is characterized It has high concentrations of linoleic acid, which activates brown fat cells filled with mitochondrial points, increasing oxygen consumption followed by increased burning of excess fat, and thus decreasing weight and agility, It is worth noting that this fatty acid has become a major component in high fitness capsules and has appeared in a large number of pharmacies.

26 - There is no doubt that the process of maintaining weight is no less important than the process of weight loss, For weight control, if you want to eat any kind of candy or fruit, it is best to have it after eating the main meal three hours, With the need to be careful of fats, especially fatty meat because they contain high prices, with the excessive intake of food containing fiber because it facilitates the disposal of body deposits, with the division of meals one to four or five meals since the multiple meals helps to control the weight of the body because The body consumes after each meal a number of calories to digest each meal, which in turn helps to lose weight. Be careful not to eat more than one type of fatty food in a meal. Body weight must be monitored by body weight every week so that the increase in the body weight can be known and can always be easily eliminated at first without having to resort to another diet to control weight.

27 - Although the internationally recognized rehydrate drugs help to reduce weight she is now safe and has said her side effects from the past, however. They should be handled with caution for the following reasons:

1-Drugs that work on the nervous system, which were used in the past such as duration "Amphetamine", which works on the center of hunger in the brain and reduces appetite and cause high-pressure Blood and nervousness are too dangerous to use now after the advent of diet drugs Modern safe.

2-Drugs that work on the center of satiety and not the center of hunger, which gives a sense of satiety because of the substance " Sibutramine " which is safe to use for up to six months and help to maintain weight but prohibited use in the case of high blood pressure, only if organized and controlled with The doctor also prohibits the use of drugs with depression and is used mainly for people with obesity and its complications, such as diabetes, high cholesterol and arthritis, and to prevent a permanent sense of hunger. These drugs can reduce 10% of the patient's body weight within a year.

3-Weeds and diuretics may have some serious side effects on public health, such as water and salt loss, leading to a decline in blood circulation.

4-However, the following other diet drugs may be used safely, including but not limited :

1- Drugs that work on the digestive system, such as orlistat, which acts as a barrier to the digestive enzymes of fat from the pancreas.

2- Chromium is one of the minerals needed by the body in small amounts to stimulate the biological processes to help to fully consume intracellular sugar.

3-Medications contain the substance of metformin and have an effect in reducing appetite and increasing the burning of sugar in Tissue.

4- Chitosan is extracted from oysters and works to absorb fat as a sponge in stomach.

5- Drugs containing the substance "hydroxy citric acid" is a substance found in vinegar apple will reduce the conversion of carbohydrates to fat.

28 - When dieting systems are applied, avoid junk food or so-called Food is "Tai chai" although it is still the favorite food when most individuals the family has almost become the main food for many families inside and outside the home high-calorie fast food such as:

- Sandwiches and Beef Sandwiches Burger, Sauce Sandwiches, Pizza, Pies, McDonald's Meats & Cheese Sandwiches, Kentucky chicken sandwich, and French fries with soft drinks or fruit juices preserved or sweetened.

The danger of these fast food is that children, adolescents and women are the most age groups to be addressed until they become part of their daily lives, which opens the areas of risk of dealing represented in the incidence of many chronic diseases associated with the treatment, for example, but not limited to:

1-High blood pressure because it is rich in sodium in the salt table.

2-The incidence of constipation and indigestion not contain the fruit and the authorities rich in dietary fiber necessary for the work of the intestines and facilitate the process of output and they are eaten hastily without chewing well.

3-The incidence of overweight, early injury heart disease and atherosclerosis and diabetes, especially cancer of the colon and breast, the incidence of diseases of the age because of the high content of fats, proteins and sugars and lack of contents of dietary fiber and vitamins and minerals useful, resulting in the accumulation of fat and sugars in the body.

4-The incidence of food poisoning, especially in the summer because of the lack of these fast food often for health conditions that prevent pollution of salmonella bacteria and increase the chances of transporting dangerous bacteria to consumers.

29 – It is not enough to resort to obese or overweight to diet drugs to get rid of excess weight because, as noted by the World Health Organization, there are key factors dealing with obesity beside diet drugs, the most important:

1-The behavior of the obese patient and his dietary culture: This includes not eating during reading or Watching television and not going to food when faced with stress or critical situations.

As well as fix dates to eat meals and quantities and try to eat before feeling hungry.

2-The need to follow an integrated diet includes all nutrients to maintain public health and reduce weight healthily without side effects.

3-Follow an appropriate sports program without exaggeration to avoid hypoglycemia, dizziness, and headaches.

30 – It is worth mentioning that there is a syndrome between weight gain and the incidence of atherosclerosis, coronary insufficiency, and stroke and stroke and these risk factors are called metabolic syndrome and perhaps the most serious and most important of these factors is the waist circumference, which indicates obesity.

Therefore, when applying dietetic systems, we should not overlook the following recommendations developed by the American Heart Organization and the International Heart Institute, which indicated that there are three or more of the following risk factors for diagnosis of coronary artery disease:

1-If the waist circumference is greater than 88 cm.

2-High triglyceride (blood triglycerides) in blood for 150 mg / 100 ml blood.

3-Low HDL cholesterol of 40.

4-High blood pressure about 140/90 .

5-The high fasting sugar level of 100 mg / 100 ml blood.

Based on the above, it is necessary to apply weight reduction diet to lose weight to the ideal weight of the body with the need to exercise for half an hour a day at least three times a week with a focus on eating healthy and completely eating saturated fats in eating, which reduces the incidence of deficiency Coronary arteries, control of high blood pressure and control of blood sugar by taking regular medication with follow-up doctor specializing in the case of high blood pressure or blood sugar.

31 – It should not be forgotten that obesity is considered the epidemic of the current century in terms of its massive spread throughout the world and in terms of the seriousness of the public health of the human being because it is accompanied by many chronic diseases such as hypertension, diabetes and atherosclerosis and heart and lung, Are a direct cause of death.

Excess obesity is said to increase BMI from 35, while people with normal obesity have a BMI of between 30 and 35.

Food diet alone is not useful in the treatment of obesity because the only treatment is the surgical treatment, which is new in the surgery of the stomach is divided into or belt two types of surgery is a reduction of the stomach by stapling and other type is the conversion of stomach and stapling stomach or stomach belt is a safe operation For most obese patients who do not suffer from a craving for sweets. The process of converting the stomach is a staple of the stomach and then converted into the small intestine and is suitable only for patients with obesity, who suffer from binge sweets.

These surgical procedures can be performed using traditional surgical methods or using a surgical endoscope. The advantages of using the surgical endoscope are the feeling of the less pain after the surgery and the patient's stay in the hospital is less and he can return to work within a few days and the surgical endoscope is not accompanied by surgical scarring after traction As in traditional surgical methods.

32 - Women use yoga to lose weight as the ideal way to maintain

weight and eliminate excess pounds without refraining from eating. Yoga is a philosophy that helps meditation, clarity of mind, closeness to God, good health and peace of mind.
Strengthen the lung muscle and improve its functions, as well as it helps to reduce the incidence of heart disease and inflammation of joints and limbs. Yoga also helps eliminate rashes and also helps prevent the diseases of the times.

 Therefore, the Yoga diet is a magical diet with many health, therapeutic and nutritional benefits because it facilitates the process of digestion and regulates blood circulation and treatment of diabetes, hypertension, arteriosclerosis, and obesity.

33 - It is important to note that frequent diet leads to obesity and increase fat cells because the weight fluctuation repeated during repeated cycles of weight loss in the case of dietary diet is the final outcome of the increase in weight because many of those who succeed in the short term in the elimination of excess weight fail To maintain what they have achieved in the long term to return their bodies to the first state.

In the sense that weight swings make it difficult to respond to diet later, and that food restriction and frequent food excess lead to an imbalance in the body's handling of energy, which in turn facilitates the incidence of obesity. As well as a structural change occurs in the body to increase the proportion of fatty tissue to the muscle tissue in the body weight, which makes the weight more and the body's willingness to give away fatless.

This change may in some way restore the ability to divide. Recent research has shown an increase in the number of fat cells equivalent to 5% during the diet period, 5% During the weight recovery period, each cycle of weight swings increases the number of fat cells by 10 % .

This means that repeated diet eventually leads to obesity and that people who have not repeated diet are the final outcome of their weight better.

34 - People should not be deceived by slimming drugs because they cause malnutrition due to the lack of mineral salts as well as the occurrence of liver lipid and cirrhosis. If it is the type that works directly on the brain, it reduces appetite but it damages the heart valves And cause high blood pressure and may cause many deaths, although it is the type that works on the stomach by filling a large space within the containment of fibers absorb water and swelling occur, such as fruits, pectin, oats and oatmeal preparations and some drugs that inhibit the work of digestive enzymes Reducing the absorption of carbohydrates, and some drugs that inhibit the work of digestive enzymes and reduce the absorption of carbohydrates, and some drugs that reduce the activity of the enzyme responsible for digestion of fat.

35 - It is important to note that when preparing food diet systems, foods containing selenium, such as shrimp, peanuts, nuts, fish, liver, chicken breasts, meat, eggs, yogurt, grains, garlic, and bread should be included.

 The lack of selenium leads to inflammation of the muscles, joints, hypertension and heart disorders Anemia, hypothyroidism, low efficiency of the body's immune system and inability to get rid of the toxicity of heavy metals such as lead and mercury.

Selenium is involved in the synthesis of 11 important proteins in addition to the formation of the enzyme antioxidant.

36 - Tilbina, which is made from whole barley flour, is made of bran and made of thin soup in the milk texture by adding a tablespoon of barley flour to a glass of water or milk and stirring it with fire. This is very important food in the case of preparing diet systems to contain barley grains on fibers of nutritional value And high protein and amino acids, mineral salts such as potassium, magnesium and vitamins of the many antioxidants, as well as distinguished by the presence of natural melatonin, which decreases with age, which is important for the prevention of heart disease and antihypertensive, The glucan found in barley helps reduce blood cholesterol, increase body immunity, delay the onset of aging and increase urine administration.

In addition, barley grain is one of the most important sources of chromium, which increases the effectiveness of insulin. Blood and reduce its complications, also helps to produce an anti-aging hormone DHEA.

37 - Usually, many people drink soda water after eating fatty meals in the belief that it helps digestion and this concept is wrong because it causes indigestion and not the reverse because it contains the substance of bicarbonate, an alkaline substance enters the sodium in the composition and when eating soda water after food, bicarbonate combine with acid The hydrochloric acid in the stomach is composed of sodium chloride, which causes the reduction of, hydrochloric acid in the stomach, which plays an important role in digestion.

Digestive enzymes cause digestion. Digestive enzymes lose digestion because they work only in acidic medium. The water changes from the middle of the stomach to the alkaline medium, and the carbonated water when activated by bicarbonate with the gastric acid hydrochloric acid results in this reaction. Open the doors of the stomach to market food before digestion into the intestine, resulting in indigestion and problems in the absorption process.

This means that the intake of carbonated water increases the sodium chloride in the body, resulting in increased blood pressure and increased alkalinity of the blood, causing general weakness and insomnia. As the calories are high in the water, drinking it increases weight and causes obesity.

Soft drinks with natural fruit juices when making food regimes.

It is worth mentioning that soda drinks consist mainly of sugar, carbon gas, colored materials, disinfectants and acidic substances, all of which have no health value at all, which explains the increased incidence of fractures among children who drink too much soda to replace milk milk that carries the calcium needed to build Solid and durable bones capable of increasing endurance.

In addition to this, the habit of drinking soda water eliminates another good food and water leakage, water makes blood better, soda drinks are quite the opposite, leading to blood lift resulting in the formation of clots responsible for heart and brain crises later.

It should not be overlooked that a large proportion of adolescents consume about 800 milligrams of caffeine daily by drinking carbonated water, although the allowed daily dose should not exceed 65 mg only.

38 - The methods and types of regimes to reduce weight are

countless, including the use of olive oil and local water sugar, take a teaspoon of olive oil a day with a cup of hot water local sweet teaspoon of sugar between meals works to reduce body weight, depending on this method to subject the body For the process of burning calories generating energy.

39 - The application and application of dieting regimens takes

into account the increased intake of fruits and vegetables Whole grains and low-fat dairy products while reducing diets rich in calories, saturated fat, salt and sugar, and avoid eating caffeine-containing products due to their harmful effects as they are one of the factors that help to get headaches and depression.

The need to avoid eating chips of chips, corn, sweets containing sugar, iced tea and drinks made from poor fruit juices to meet the increasing number of children and adolescents because of their intake of these foods.

40 - In the application and application of balanced diet diets, the dimension should be taken away from the low-carbohydrate and high-carbohydrate regimes, the one-food-based regimens, and the less-than-analogized regimens because of these regimens Many of the risks that we mention, for example, but not limited to :

1-Its negative effects on the work and functions of all organs of the body.

2-Side effects such as constipation, diarrhea, anemia or menstrual cycle disorders.

3-Recurrence leads to increased body fat and lack of muscle tissue. Increase uric acid resulting in gout.

4-The occurrence of dryness in the skin and sagging especially in the abdomen.

5-Increase the proportion of cholesterol in the blood as a result of the movement of fat stocks causing gallstones.

6-The incidence of headaches, physical fatigue, tension, nervousness, and rapid emotion.

Chapter 4

You should eat some vegetables, fruits, foods and drinks within a week to get good results.

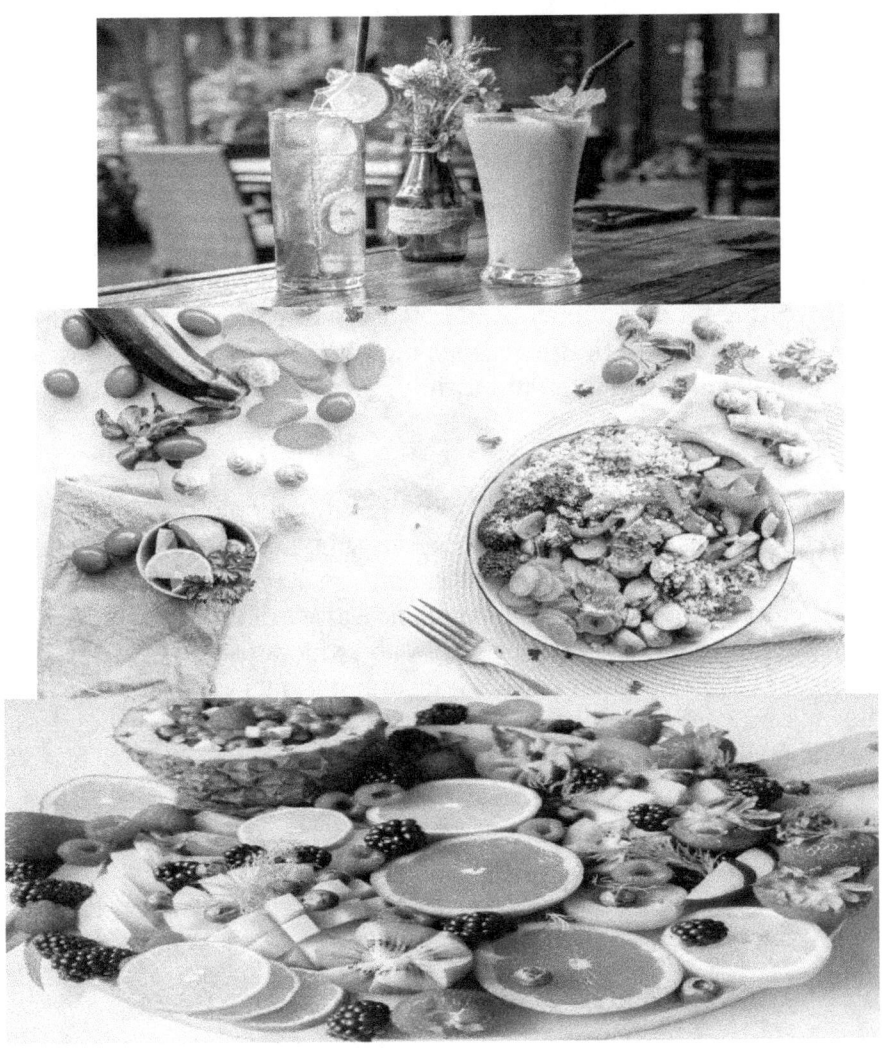

Chapter 5

The detailed feeding system consists of Breakfast, lunch and dinner.

Guide to meals for a week

The diet is defined as the food, the drink consumed by someone, depending on the physical and mental conditions that determine the nature of the food, and may be a diet consisting of a special group, or specific food and drink, for reasons including improving health, or access to healthy weight , And ideally, be within a plan, or a daily program.

The diet plays an important role in protecting people from chronic diseases such as heart disease, blood vessels, diabetes, cancer, and some cases associated with obesity, and can stay away from the risk of developing these diseases through a healthy diet that includes: Fruits, legumes, nuts, grains, along with reducing salt, sugar, choosing unsaturated fats instead of saturated fats to reduce trans fats, taking care to reduce the amount of fat consumed in general, I've planned for you and chose you diet For seven days consists of:

-The principal day relies upon eating new organic product aside from bananas since it contains numerous calories, and never takes apples rather than espresso, since they will be on caution, and be mindful so as to partition your day into 4-6 servings of natural product. Try not to drink dark tea, espresso, sugars or other non-characteristic sugars and drink a lot of water.

Breakfast: omelets with various vegetables, fried with butter or coconut oil.
Lunch: Cheese burger with no additives, served with vegetables and salsa sauce.
Dinner: Yogurt cooked with grapes with blue berries and a handful of almonds.

-The second day of slimming down relies upon crisp vegetables of any amount you incline toward. Avoid any meat items. In the event that you need to eat cooked vegetables, don't include in excess of a teaspoon of oil. You can possibly include herbs and common flavors while planning vegetables; you can likewise eat vegetables as plate of mixed greens, and remember to drink a lot of water.

Breakfast: Meat with eggs.

Lunch: salmon with butter and vegetables.

Dinner: Cheese burger with no additives, served with vegetables.

-The third day of the eating routine relies upon eating any measure of products of the soil for the duration of the day and recall that you ought not to drink dark tea or sodas all through the framework days. You can likewise eat the accompanying vegetable soup as a dietary enhancement since it gives you salt, water, protein, vitality and different supplements. Elements of vegetable soup: water, huge onions, green peppers, tomatoes with cabbage, celery, herbs, and flavors. You can likewise include different vegetables, for example, corn, green beans, turnips, and cauliflower, yet maintain a strategic distance from the beans since they contain high calories.

Breakfast: Eggs and vegetables fried in butter or coconut oil.

Lunch: grilled chicken with vegetables.

Dinner: shrimp salad with some olive oil.

-The fourth day of suppers relies upon eating bananas and skimmed milk at breakfast (limit of 8 bananas) on the grounds that the blend of milk and bananas at breakfast gives you a great deal of vitality. For supper, you can eat vegetable soup a similar route as on the third day.

Breakfast: egg omelets and fried vegetables in butter or coconut oil.

Lunch: a piece of meat and assorted vegetables.

Dinner: juice with coconut milk, or berries, or almonds, or protein powder.

-The fifth day relies upon the eating regimen: you can eat meat (new meat as much as 300 grams) and tomatoes (greatest 2 tomatoes for each feast). On the off chance that you are a vegan, you can substitute hamburger with a measure of rice. Drink a lot of water throughout the day.

Breakfast: meat and eggs.

Lunch: Steak with veg.

Dinner: chicken salad with some olive oil.

- The 6th day of consuming less calories relies upon eating lean meat with six tomatoes. You can likewise include crisp or cooked vegetables. For veggie   lovers, they can supplant rice with meat.

Breakfast: egg omelets and various vegetables.

Lunch: meat balls with vegetables.

Dinner: White yogurt with berries, coconut flakes, and a handful of walnuts.

-Relies upon the seventh day in the eating regimen, you ought to eat dark colored rice and organic product juice for breakfast. For nourishment and supper, you can eat any sort of vegetables in any amount. You can likewise eat organic product squeezes by lunch and supper.

Breakfast: meat and eggs.

Lunch: grilled chicken wings with some raw spinach on the side.

Dinner: juice with coconut milk, with a little creamy, protein powder flavored with chocolate and berries.

Notwithstanding the seven-day solid feast framework, we include a choice of formulas that can be utilized in your thinning program.

Chapter 6

More than 30 natural healthy recipes for fast weight loss.

-The lemon recipe:

A study published in the Journal of Chemistry and Nutrition has shown the effective role of lemon in the weight loss because it contains polyphones, which have been shown to reduce the weight of a group of high-fat diets. On the human, however, there are many experiments that have shown the importance of lemon in slimming.

Mix a glass of lemon juice and two cups of water. Eat this mixture every morning on your stomach to burn a large percentage of fat.

-Apple and Honey Cider:

Mix a tablespoon of honey, two tablespoons of apple cider vinegar and a cup of warm water, and drink three times a day before eating the three main meals.

-Apple vinegar recipe:

Apple cider vinegar is used in weight loss recipes, so that one tablespoon of natural vinegar is placed in a glass of water, stirred and then drunk in 3 batches daily, 30 minutes before meals. This method is followed for several weeks. With a teaspoon of cinnamon ground in a glass of water, and a little honey can be added. [Although apple cider vinegar contains fiber that increases satiety, and despite the role, it plays in accelerating metabolism, some experts like Catherine Zaritsky of Mayo Clinic They do not believe in vinegar as a recipe for cutting Weight, and do not recognize its impact on the process of acting.

-The recipe for green tea:

Green tea has the potential to burn fat, promote metabolism, and contains large amounts of polyuns, as well as antioxidants, according to the University of Maryland Medical (UMMC), a group of researchers have discovered that a substance called caffeine found in green tea reduces weight well , Especially for quail people, so that
this article is burning fat in the body is recommended to drink green tea after eating.

-Other recipes for fast weight loss:

Cucumber and peppermint: Place in the food preparation a number of fresh mint leaves, cucumber, half a cup of water, and small vinaigrette of lemon juice, and drink a cup of the mixture every morning on an empty stomach.

Ginger and peppermint: Cut a piece of ginger and put in boiling water, add a few fresh mint leaves, put the mixture on the fire and let it boil for 30 minutes. Then,
remove it from the fire, leave it to cool and then cook. Every meal.

Cumin and garlic: Put a bowl on the fire and add two cups of water, a teaspoon of cumin powder and nine cloves of garlic, and leave the mixture boiling for 15 minutes, then lift the fire and let it cool, then put it in the food preparation and mix well, and drink A cup of this mixture every morning after waking up straight from sleep.

Cumin and Cinnamon: Bring a cup of boiled water, add a teaspoon of cinnamon powder and three tablespoons of cumin powder and half a lemon, and
then cool the mixture and drink it after each meal.

Mermia: Add a large tablespoon of sage leaves to a cup of boiling water, then put the mixture on the fire and let it boil for 15 minutes, and drink this drink every evening and before going to sleep.

Milk: It is rich in calcium, and has a role in the elimination of fat in fat cells, so the addition of milk to the daily diet accelerates weight loss.

Black Bean & Rice Enchiladas

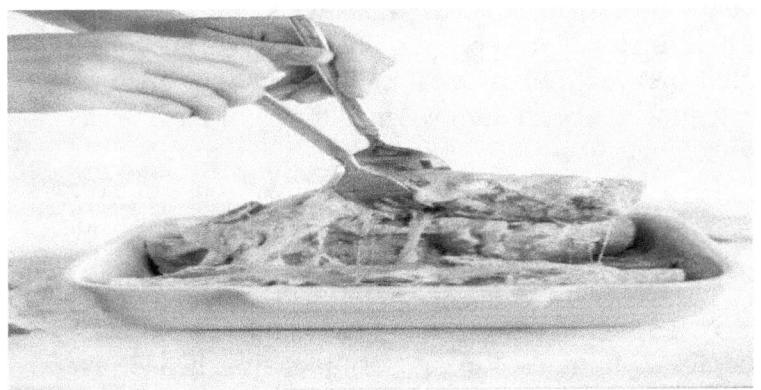

Ingredients:

-1 Tablespoon olive oil
-1 Green pepper, chopped
-1 Medium onion, chopped
-3 Garlic cloves, minced
-1 Can (15 ounces) dark beans, washed and drained
-1 Can (14-1/2 ounces) diced tomatoes and green chilies
-1/4 Cup Picante sauce
-1 Tablespoon chili powder
-1 Teaspoon ground cumin
-1/4 Teaspoon crushed red pepper flakes
-2 Cups cooked brown rice
-8 Flour tortillas (6 inches), warmed
-1 Cup of salsa
-1 Cup shredded reduced-fat cheddar cheese
-3 Tablespoons chopped fresh cilantro leaves

Method:

Preheat stove to 350°. In an expansive nonstick skillet, heat oil over medium warmth. Include green pepper, onion, and garlic; sauté until delicate. Include next six fixings; heat to the point of boiling. Decrease heat; stew, revealed until warmed through. Include rice, cook 5 minutes longer.

Spoon an adjusted 1/2 measure of rice blend down focus of every tortilla. Crease sides over topping and move off. Spot crease side down in a 13x9-in. heating dish covered with cooking shower. Spoon remaining rice blend along sides of the dish. Top tortillas with salsa.

Heat, secured, for 25 minutes. Reveal, sprinkle with cheddar. Heat until cheddar is softened, 2-3 minutes longer. Sprinkle with cilantro before serving.

Chicken Soup and Ginger

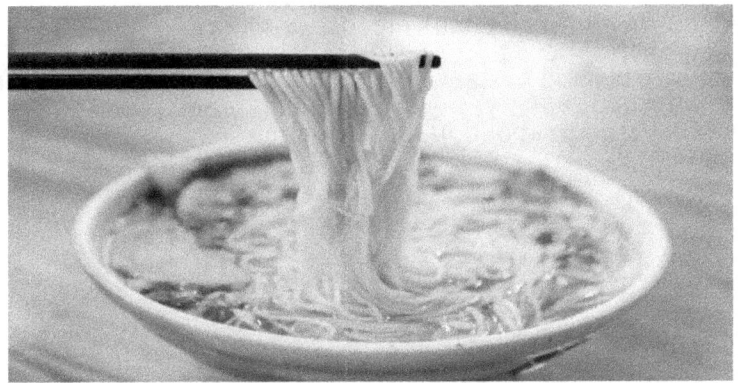

Ingredients:

-1 Pound boneless skinless chicken bosoms, cubed

-2 Medium carrots, shredded

-3 Tablespoons sherry or diminished sodium chicken juices

-2 Tablespoons rice vinegar

-1 Tablespoon reduced-sodium soy sauce

-2 To 3 Teaspoons minced fresh gingerroot

-1/4 Teaspoon pepper

-6 Cups reduced-sodium chicken broth

-1 Cup water

-2 Cups fresh snow peas, halved

-2 Ounces uncooked angel hair pasta, broken into thirds

Method:

In a 5-qt. slow cooker, combine the first nine ingredients. Cook, covered, on low until chicken is tender, 3-4 hours.

Stir in snow peas and pasta. Cook, covered, on low until snow peas and pasta are tender, about 30 minutes longer.

Mushroom mushrooms wraps

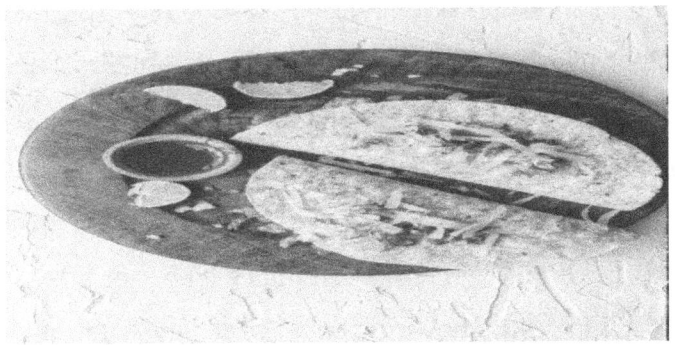

Ingredients:

-4 Teaspoons sesame or canola oil, divided

-4 Large eggs, lightly beaten

-1/2 Pound sliced fresh mushrooms

-1 Package (12 ounces) broccoli coleslaw mix

-2 Garlic cloves, minced

-2 Teaspoons minced fresh gingerroot

-2 Tablespoons rice vinegar

-2 Tablespoons reduced-sodium soy sauce

-2 Teaspoons Sriracha chili sauce

-1 Cup fresh bean sprouts

-1/2 Cup hoi sin sauce

-10 Flour tortillas (6 inches), warmed

-6 Green onions, sliced

Method:

In a substantial nonstick skillet, heat 1 teaspoon oil over medium warmth. Pour in eggs; cook and mix until eggs are thickened and no fluid egg remains. Expel from skillet.

In a similar skillet, heat remaining oil over medium-high warmth. Include mushrooms; cook and blend until delicate. Include coleslaw blend, garlic, and ginger; cook 1-2 minutes longer or until slaw is fresh delicate. In a little bowl, blend vinegar, soy sauce, and bean stew sauce; add to the dish. Mix in sprouts and eggs; heat through. Spread around 2 teaspoons hoi sin sauce over every tortilla to inside 1/4 in. of edges. Layer with 1/2 glass vegetable blend and around 1 tablespoon green onion. Move up firmly.

Spring vegetables

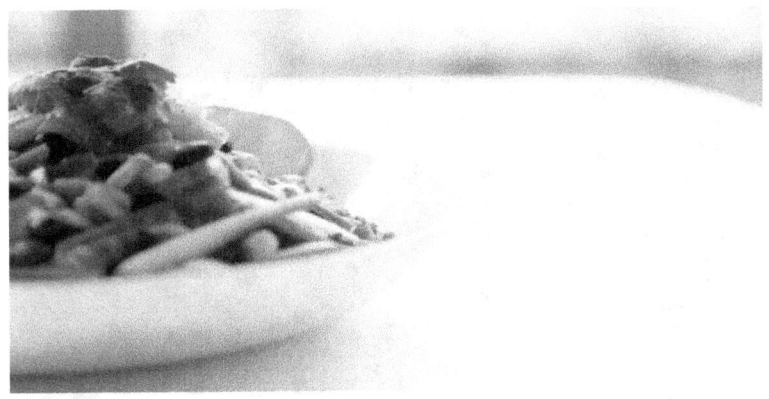

Ingredients:

-2 oz dry entier grain farfelue pesta

-2 tsp olive oil

-1/2 Cup artichoke hearts

-1/4 Cup sliced red onion

-1/4 Cup peas

-1 Tbsp slashed new mint

Method:

Cook pasta as coordinated and hurl with oil, vegetables, and mint.
Season with salt and pepper to taste.
Per serving: 370 cal

Soft pork and soft vegetables

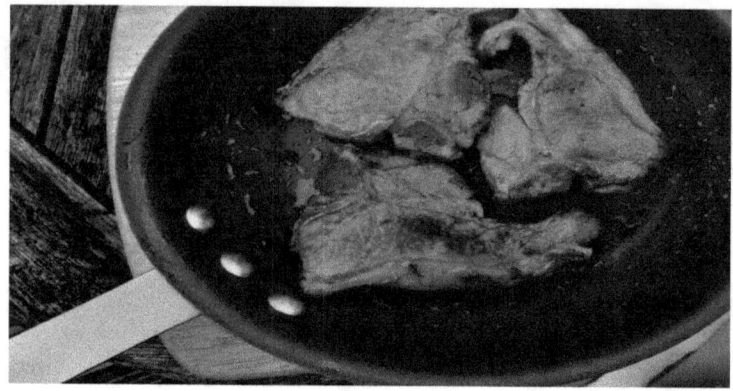

Ingredients:

-1 Pork tenderloin (4 oz)

-1 Container steamed green beans

-2 Tbsp cut almonds

-1 Baked sweet potato

Method:

Season pork with salt and pepper, singe in an ovenproof skillet covered with cooking shower and exchange to a 450°F stove for 15 minutes. Cut and present with green beans finished with almonds and sweet potato.

Per serving: 370 cal.

Light Lasagna

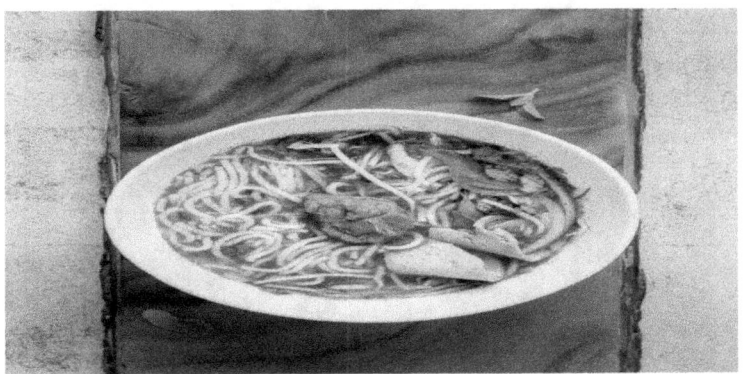

Ingredients:

-1/2 Cup cooked whole-wheat spaghett
-1/4 Cup part-skim ricott
-1/2 Tsp crushed red chili flake
-1 Coleman Natural Mild Italian Chicken Sausage link, cooked
-2 Cups spinach

Method:

Consolidate pasta, ricotta, and bean stew drops, at that point disintegrate hotdog on top. Include spinach, and let shrink.

Eggs and potatoes

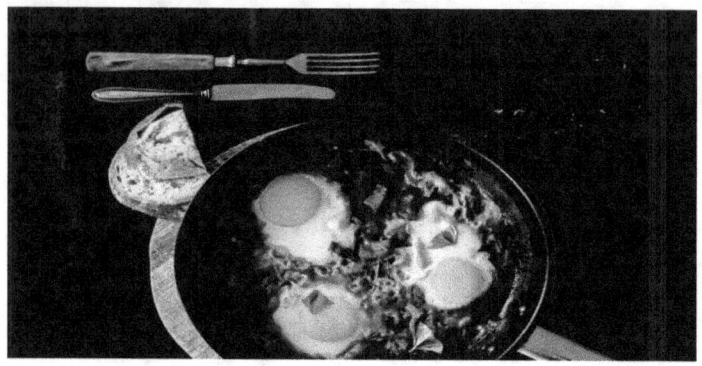

Ingredients:

-3 Tablespoons butter
-1 Pounds red potatoes, chopped
-1/4 Cup minced fresh parsley
-2 Garlic cloves, minced
-3/4 Teaspoon kosher salt
-1/8 Teaspoon peppe
-3 Large eggs
-1/2 Cup shredded extra-sharp cheddar cheese

Method:

Preheat broiler to 400°. In a 10-in. cast-iron or another ovenproof skillet, heat spread over medium-high warmth. Include potatoes; cook and blend until brilliant darker and delicate. Blend in parsley, garlic, salt, and pepper. With the back of a spoon, make four wells in the potato blend; break the eggs.

Prepare until egg whites are totally set and yolks start to thicken yet are not hard, 9-11 minutes. Sprinkle with cheddar; prepare until cheddar is dissolved, 1 minute.

Grilled Salmon in the compartments

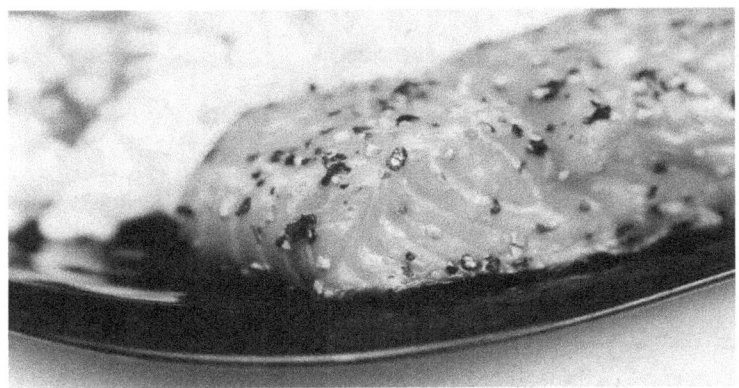

Ingredients:

-2 Tablespoons olive oil
-1 Tablespoon reduced-sodium soy sauce
-2 Teaspoons Dijon mustard
-1/4 Teaspoon dried minced garlic
-2 Salmon fillets (5 ounces each)

Method:

In a little bowl, consolidate the oil, soy sauce, mustard, and garlic. Empty portion of the marinade into a shallow dish. Add the salmon and swing to coat. Spread; refrigerate for 30 minutes. Spread and refrigerate remaining marinade.
Channel fish and dispose of marinade. On a lubed flame broil rack, barbecue salmon, secured, over high warmth until fish drops effectively with a fork,
5-10 minutes. Sprinkle with saved marinade.

Juicer juice with avocado

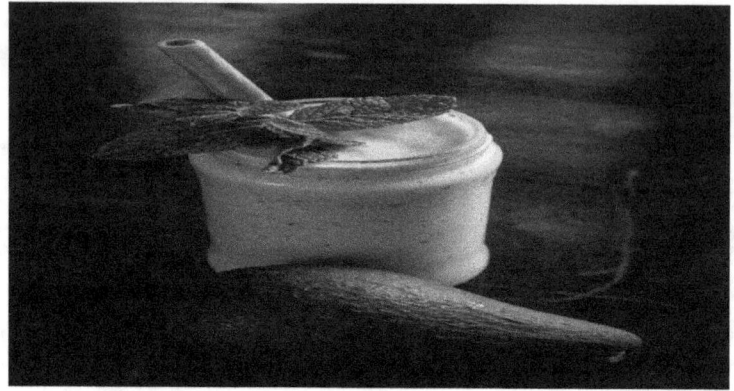

Ingredients:

-Cup of water -1/2 1

-Avocado 1

-1 Watercress pack

-1/2 Cup honey bee

Method:

Mix the watercress with the water in the blender.

Crispy avocado and cut and oily.

And after the guest honey bee and continue to mix.

Vegetarian Black Bean Pasta

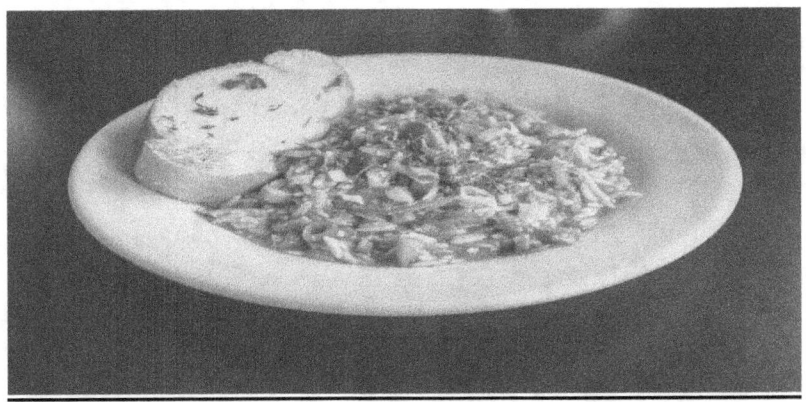

Ingredients:

-9 Ounces uncooked whole wheat fettuccine
-1 Tablespoon olive oil
-1 -3/4 cups sliced baby Portobello mushrooms
-1 Garlic clove, minced
-1 Can (15 ounces) black beans, rinsed and drained
-1 Can (14-1/2 ounces) diced tomatoes, untrained
-1 Teaspoon dried rosemary, crushed
-1/2 Teaspoon dried oregano
-2 Cups fresh baby spinach

Method:

Cook fettuccine as per bundle headings. In the interim, in an extensive skillet, heat oil over medium-high warmth. Include mushrooms; cook and mix 4-6 minutes or until delicate. Include garlic, cook 1 minute longer.

Blend in dark beans, tomatoes, rosemary and oregano; heat through. Mix in spinach until withered. Channel fettuccine; add to bean blend and hurl to consolidate.

Curried Rice & Noodles

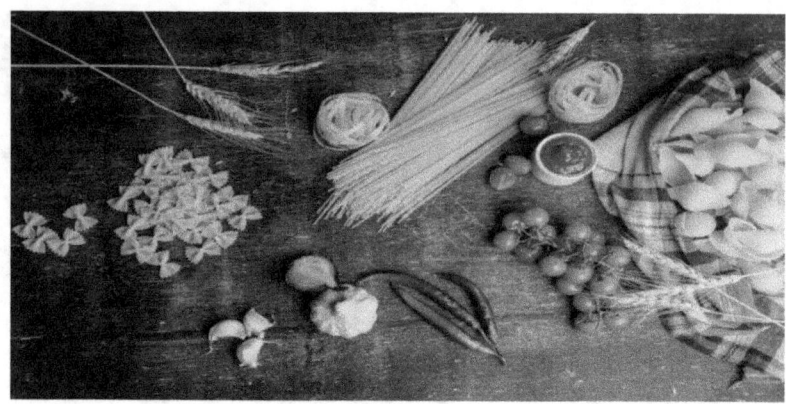

Ingredients:

-2 Ounces uncooked multigrain angel hair pasta, broken into 1- to 2-inch piece
-2 Large eggs, lightly beaten
-1 Tablespoon canola oil
-1 Yellow summer squash, sliced
-1 Small sweet red pepper, chopped
-2 Garlic cloves, minced
-2 Teaspoons curry powder
-1/2 Teaspoon ground ginger
-1/4 Teaspoon crushed red pepper flakes
-1 Package (8-1/2 ounces) ready-to-serve basmati rice
-2 Tablespoons reduced-sodium soy sauce
-1 Tablespoon lime juice
-1 Teaspoon sesame oil
-2 Green onions, thinly sliced
-1/2 Cup chopped cashews

Method:

In a little pan, cook pasta as per bundle bearings; channel and cool. In the meantime, place an extensive nonstick skillet covered with cooking splash over medium warmth. Pour in eggs; cook and blend until eggs are thickened and no fluid egg remains. Expel from a dish. In same skillet, heat canola oil over medium-high warmth. Include squash, red pepper, and garlic; pan sear 2-3 minutes or until squash is fresh delicate. Mix in curry powder, ginger and pepper drops. Include rice and pasta, sprinkle with soy sauce, lime juice, and sesame oil. Warmth through, hurling to consolidate. Blend in green onions, cashews, and cooked eggs.

Hearty White Bean Soup

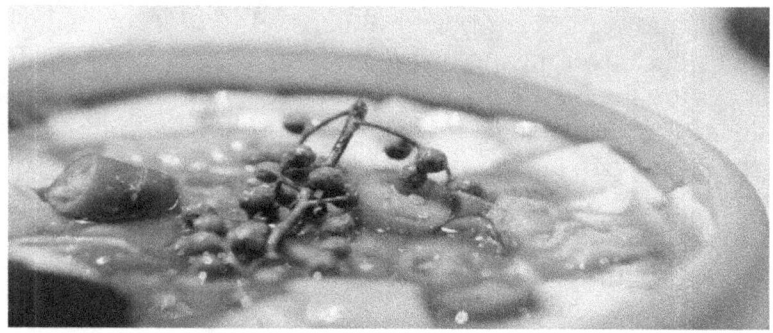

Ingredients:

-1 Tablespoon olive oil
-1 Medium potato, peeled and cut into 1/2-inch cubes
-2 Medium carrots, chopped
-1 Medium onion, chopped
-2 Celery ribs, chopped
-1 Medium zucchini, chopped
-1 Teaspoon finely chopped seeded jalapeno pepper
-1 Can (15-1/2 ounces) navy beans, rinsed and drained
-2 To 2-1/2 cups vegetable or chicken broth
-1 Can (8 ounces) tomato sauce
-2 Tablespoons minced fresh parsley or 2 teaspoons dried parsley
flakes
-1 -1/2 Teaspoons minced fresh thyme or 1/2 teaspoon dried thyme

Method:

In a Dutch broiler, heat oil over medium-high warmth. Include
potato and carrots, cook and mix 3 minutes.
Add onion, celery, zucchini and jalapeno, cook and stir 3-4 minutes
or until vegetables are crisp-tender.
Stir in remaining ingredients, bring to a boil. Reduce heat; simmer,
covered, 12-15 minutes or until vegetables are tender.

Tomato Garlic Lentil Bowls

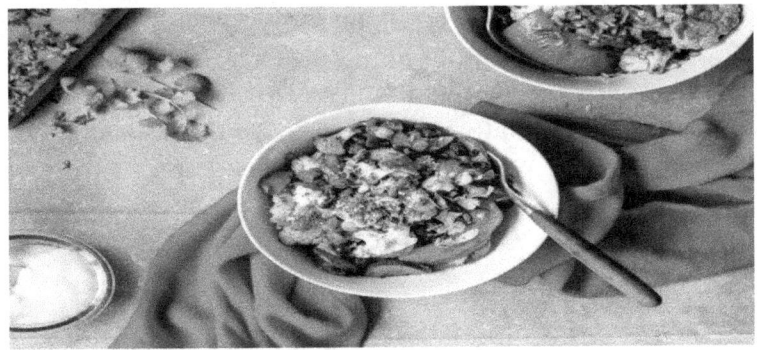

Ingredients:

-1 Tablespoon olive oil

-2 Medium onions, chopped

-4 Garlic cloves, minced

-2 Cups dried brown lentils, rinsed

-1 Teaspoon salt

-1/2 Teaspoon ground ginger

-1/2 Teaspoon paprika

-1/4 Teaspoon pepper

-3 Cups water

-1/4 Cup lemon juice

-3 Tablespoons tomato paste

-3/4 Cup fat-free plain Greek yogurt

Method:

In a huge pan, heat oil over medium-high warmth; saute onions 2 minutes. Include garlic, cook 1 minute. Mix in lentils, seasonings and water, heat to the point of boiling. Decrease heat; stew, secured, until lentils are delicate, 25-30 minutes.
Blend in lemon juice and tomato glue, heat through. Present with yogurt and, whenever wanted, tomatoes and cilantro.

White fish soup

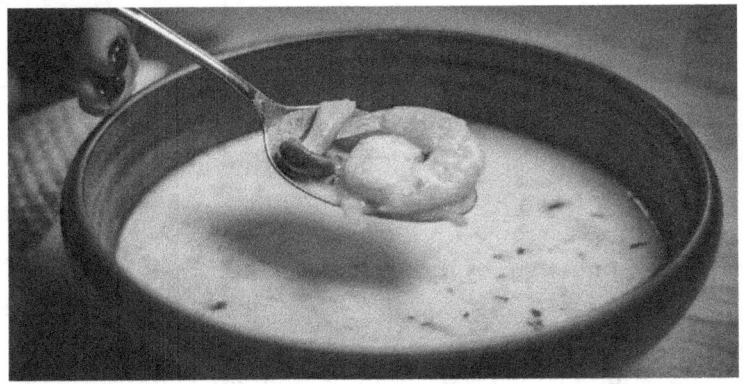

Ingredients:

-4 Pieces of fillet thickness.

-1 Potatoes cut into small cubes.

-1 Carrot
-2 Tablespoons lemon juice.

-1 Onion cut into thin wings.

-1 Teaspoon salt.

-1 Teaspoon black pepper.

-1 Laure paper.

-3 Tablespoons vegetable oil. Celery omelet clip.

-3 Cloves of crushed garlic.

-2 Tablespoons of tomato paste.

-1 Tablespoon flour.

-2 Tablespoons chopped coriander.

-2 Pieces freshly chopped tomatoes.

-Quantity of water as needed

Method:

Cut the fillet into two halves. In a pot of fire put a quantity of water and let it boil. Add the bay leaf, chopped onion, salt, and black pepper to the pot of boiling water. Add the pieces and leave them for a minute.

We bring the fish out of the pot, and then sprinkle it with the broth. In another pot put the oil, then put it on medium heat. Add the celery and garlic and stir them well, then add the flour and continue stirring. Add potatoes, tomatoes, carrots, and tomato paste, and stir well for a few minutes until the ingredients become soft.

Add the fish soup and let it cook for 15 minutes. Cut the cooked fish into small pieces, add it to the soup, and let it boil for 1 minute.

Sprinkle the soup in a deep dish, add lemon juice and sprinkle it with chopped coriander, and serve it hot.

Asian Lettuce Cups

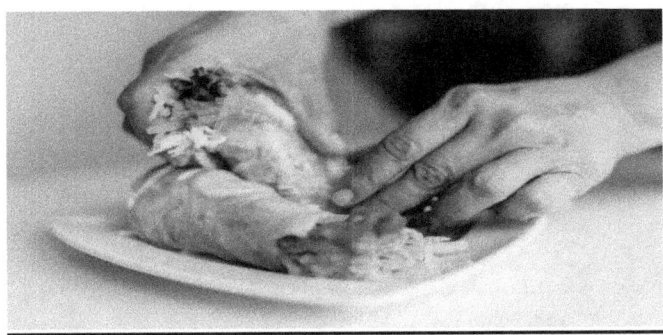

Ingredients:

-3 Tablespoons reduced-sodium soy sauce
-2 Teaspoons sugar
-2 Teaspoons sesame oil
-1 Teaspoon Thai chili sauce, optional
-1 Pound lean ground turkey
-1 Celery rib, chopped
-1 Tablespoon minced fresh gingerroot
-1 Garlic clove, minced
-1 Can (8 ounces) water chestnuts, drained and chopped
-1 Medium carrot, shredded
-2 Cups cooked brown rice
-8 Bibb or Boston lettuce leaves

Method:

In a little bowl, whisk soy sauce, sugar, sesame oil and, whenever wanted, bean stew sauce until mixed. In a substantial skillet, cook turkey and celery 6-9 minutes or until turkey is never again pink, separating turkey into disintegrates, channel.
Add ginger and garlic to turkey, cook 2 minutes. Blend in soy sauce blend, water chestnuts and carrot, cook 2 minutes longer. Blend in rice, heat through. Serve in lettuce leaves.

Broccoli Pasta Primavera

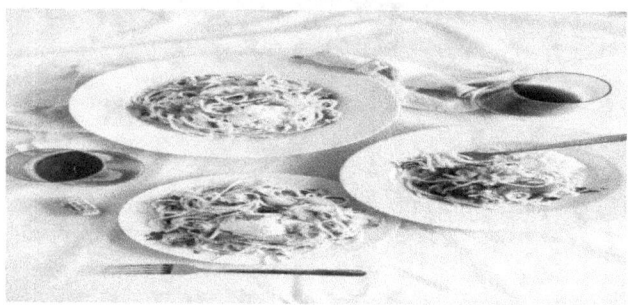

Ingredients:

-8 Ounces uncooked linguine
-1 Cup thinly sliced fresh broccoli
-1 Medium carrot, thinly sliced
-1/2 Cup sliced green onions
-1/4 Cup butter, cubed
-1-1/2 Cups sliced fresh mushrooms
-1 Garlic clove, minced
-1 Teaspoon dried basil
-1/4 Teaspoon salt and pepper salt
-6 Ounces fresh or frozen snow peas (about 2 cups), thawed
-1/4 Cup dry white wine or chicken broth
-1/4 Cup shredded Parmesan cheese

Method:

Cook linguine as indicated by bundle bearings.
In the mean time, in a huge skillet, cook the broccoli, carrot and onions in spread for 3 minutes. Include the mushrooms, garlic, basil, salt and pepper, cook 1 minute longer. Include snow peas and wine. Spread and cook for 2 minutes or until peas are fresh delicate.
Channel linguine; add to skillet and hurl to coat.
 Sprinkle with cheddar.

Tomato Soup

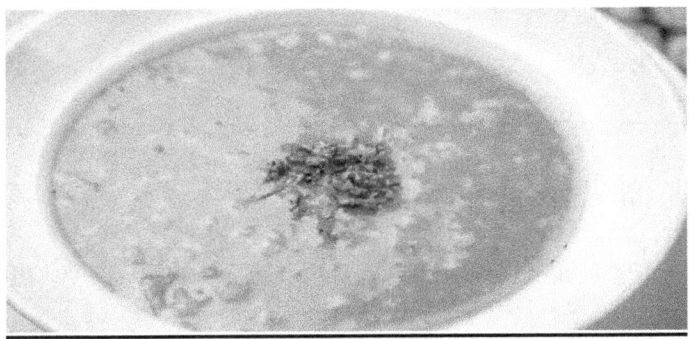

Ingredients:

-2 Teaspoons canola oil

-1/4 Cup finely chopped onion

-1/4 Cup finely chopped celery

-2 Cans (14-1/2 ounces each) diced tomatoes, untrained

-1-1/2 Cups water

-2 Teaspoons brown sugar

-1/2 Teaspoon salt

-1/2 Teaspoon dried basil

-1/4 Teaspoon dried oregano

-1/4 Teaspoon coarsely ground pepper

-Minced fresh basil, optional

Method:

In an expansive pot, heat oil over medium-high warmth. Include onion and celery, cook and blend until delicate, 2-4 minutes.
 Include remaining fixings.
Heat to the point of boiling.
Decrease heat; stew, revealed, 10 minutes to enable flavors to mix.
Puree soup utilizing a submersion blender.
Or then again cool soup somewhat and puree in bunches in a blender; come back to skillet and warmth through.
Whenever wanted, top with new minced basil.

Sun-Dried Tomato Burgers

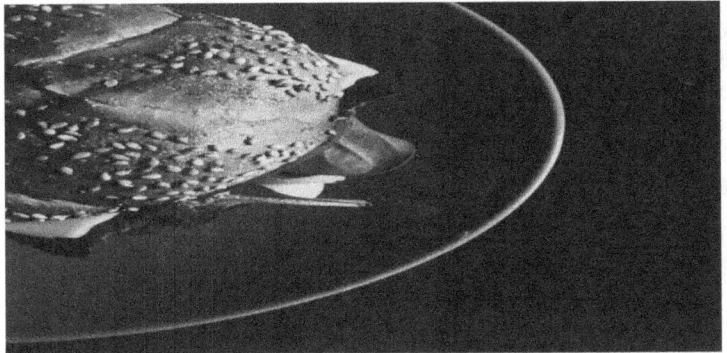

Ingredients:

-1 Large red onion
-1 Cup (4 oz) crumbled feta cheese, divided
-2/3 Cup chopped oil-packed sun-dried tomatoes
-1/4 Teaspoon salt
-1/4 Teaspoon pepper
-2 Pounds lean ground turkey
-6 Ciabatta rolls, split

Method:

Cut the onion down the middle. Finely cleave one half and meagerly cut the staying half.
Consolidate 1/2 glass feta, sun-dried tomatoes, cleaved onion, salt and pepper in a vast bowl.
 Disintegrate turkey over blend and blend well. Shape into 6 patties. Barbecue burgers, secured, over medium warmth or cook 4 in. from the warmth for 5-7 min on each side or until a thermometer peruses 165° and juices run clear.
In the interim, in a little nonstick skillet covered with cooking shower, sauté cut onion until delicate. Serve burgers with onion and remaining feta.

Hearty Lettuce Salad

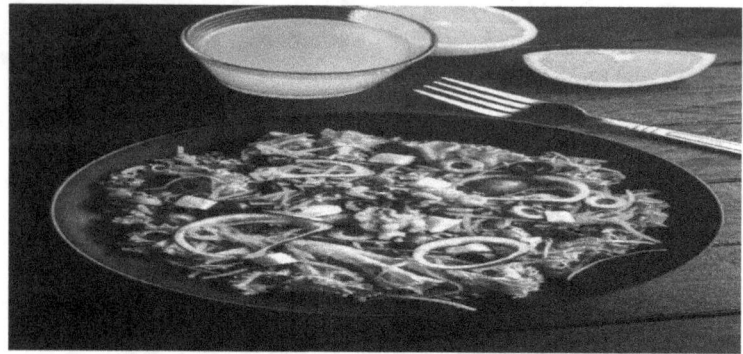

Ingredients:

-1 Cup ready-to-serve brown rice
-1 Cup frozen shelled edamame
-3 Cups spring mix salad greens
-1 /4 cup of ginger plate and reduced sesame fat
-1 Medium navel orange, peeled and sectioned
-4 Radishes, sliced
-2 Tablespoons sliced almonds, toasted

Method:

Get ready rice and edamame as per bundle bearings.
In an extensive bowl, consolidate the plate of mixed greens, rice and
edamame. Shower with plate of mixed greens dressing and hurl to
coat.
Partition serving of mixed greens blend between two plates, top with
orange portions, radishes and almonds.

Wellbeing tip :

This is a perfect nippy atmosphere essential dish plate of blended
greens when gardens are still under a layer of ice. For a heartier
adjustment, incorporate sautéed shrimp or additional rotisserie
chicken.

Fennel juice for diet

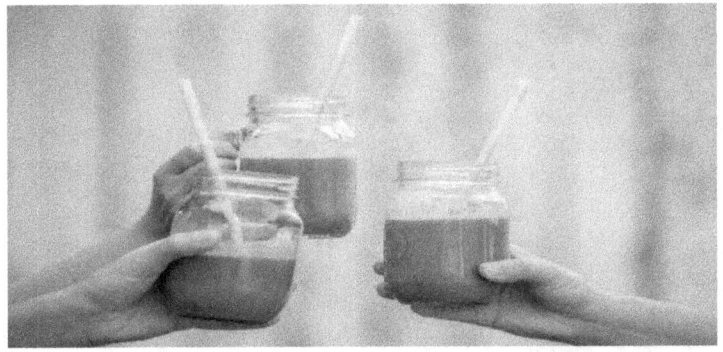

Ingredients:

-1 -1/2 Hanging small fennel seeds

-1 Water cup

-1 Cinnamon sticks

-1 Hanging small tea

Method:

Place the seeds of fennel, tea and cinnamon in boiling water for 15 minutes.

Notes:

It is recommended to drink this juice before eating a quarter of an hour to make effective effective as it is a beverage that works to fill the appetite and has a significant role in weight loss effectively.

The chicken pot is tasty

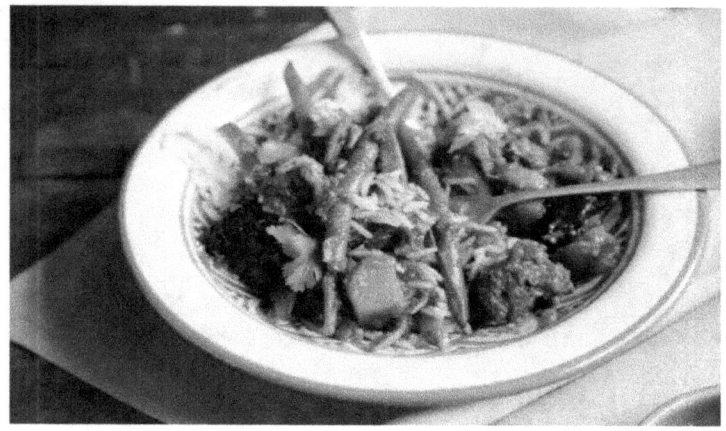

Ingredients:

-1 ½ Lbs chicken thighs (skinless, boneless)

-1 Cup brown rice (uncooked and rinsed)

-1 Tbsp olive oil

-2 ¼ Cup fat free chicken broth

-1 Large onion (finely chopped)

-2 Large carrots (diced)

-8 Oz mushrooms (sliced)

-4 Cloves garlic (minced)

-2 Tsp dried thyme

-1 Tbsp fresh lemon juice

-Salt and pepper to taste

Method:

Turn Instant Pot to "Sauté". When hot, add olive oil.

Season chicken with salt and pepper, at that point in the chicken, and darker around 3-4 minutes on each side. Expel chicken and put aside.

Deglaze the pot by pouring in ¼ cup of the chicken broth, and making sure to scrape up the browned bits on the bottom of the pan.

Add in all the chopped vegetables, and sauté for about 3 min.

Stir in the remaining broth, thyme, lemon juice and rice. Add additional salt and pepper as desired. Top with the chicken.

Turn off the "Sauté" function. Lock on lid, select the "Manual" function and set to high pressure for 20 min.

Permit to normally discharge for 10 minutes, at that point physically discharge any residual weight. Exchange chicken to plates and serve.

Leeks of chicken oil

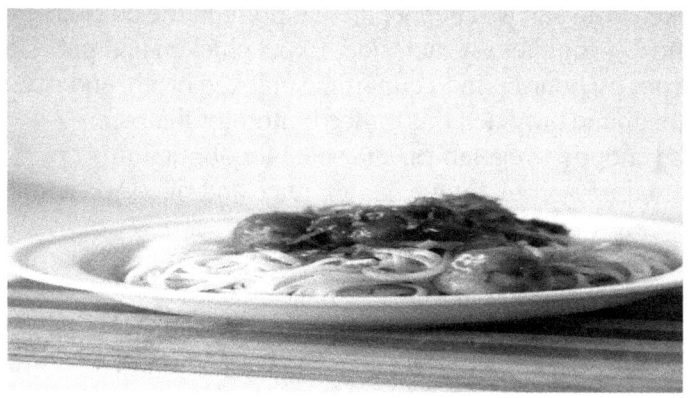

Ingredients:

-1 Pound boneless skinless chicken bosoms, cut into 1 ½ inch piec

-1 Tablespoon minced fresh rosemary, or ½ tablespoon if you are using dried rosemary
-½ Teaspoon salt
-½ Teaspoons freshly ground black pepper
-3 Teaspoons extra virgin olive oil, divided
-1 Cup chopped shallots (1½ large or three small)
-1 Clove garlic minced
-3 Tablespoons cider vinegar
-¼ Cup white wine
-1 ½ounce can diced tomatoes with their juice
-5 Pitted and chopped Kalamata olives
-1 Tablespoon capers drained
-¼ Cup fresh basil
-Pasta of your choice

Method:

Spread out chicken cuts and separation salt, pepper, and rosemary among front and back of the chicken.

Warmth a large portion of the oil in an extensive non-stick dish over medium-high warmth and cook chicken in two clusters utilizing rest of oil for the second half, around 2-3 minutes on each side per group. Put chicken aside.

Spot shallots and garlic in a container and cook for one moment until delicate. Add vinegar to deglaze the skillet.

At the point when the vinegar has dissipated, include wine, tomatoes, olives, and escapades. Cook over medium to medium-high warmth 5-8 minutes until the blend has thickened.

Add basil and return chicken to the skillet alongside any juices that have spilled out of the chicken and cook for one progressively minute.

Serve over your most loved pasta.

Carrot soup

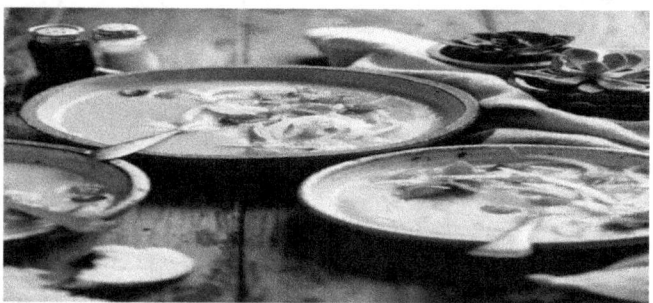

Ingredients:

-3 Cup broth chicken

-1 Hanging large starch
-1 Cup milk skimmed milk
-1 Chopped onion
-1 Kilo carrot
-1 Small suspended salt or as desired
-1 Nutmeg Brush
-1 Finely ground black pepper
-1 Hanging small corn oil

Method:

Brush with a little spray of oil and stir the onion until it changes color.
Add the carrots and stir slightly and then put the gravy and leave the mixture on medium heat until boiling.
When boiling, add salt, pepper, and nutmeg and leave on low heat until vegetables are cooked.
Mix the carrot mixture in the blender, add the starch and milk, and mix the ingredients until they are homogenous.
Bring the mixture back to the mixture and leave on low heat until it holds.

Tomato salad with mozzarella cheese

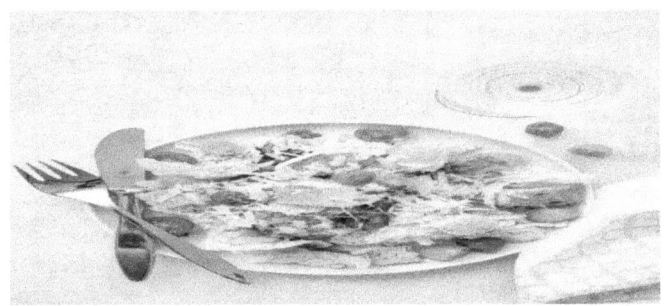

Ingredients:

-12 of basil leaves

-3 Tomatoes

-2 Cup mozzarella cheese chopped

-1 Hanging large balsamic vinegar

-1 Small hanging ground black pepper

-1 Small suspended salt

-1 Small hanging olive oil

Method:

Cut tomatoes and mozzarella cheese into slices
Then arrange tomatoes, cheese, and basil. Leaves in a circular way.
Then add salt and pepper, olive oil and a little balsamic vinegar.

Salad pasta Italians

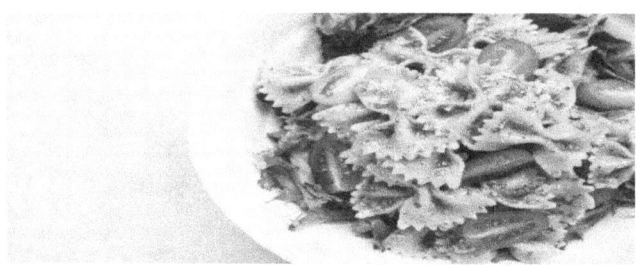

Ingredients:

-250g Papillion pasta

-Melon

-6 Cherry tomatoes
-12 Leaves of basil
-150g Of mozzarella or feta cheese
-4 Thin slices of Parma ham
-12 Black olives
-6 Tablespoons of olive oil
-Lemon/Pepper/Salt

Method:

-Step   1:   Cook the pasta 8 to 10 min.
-Step 2: cut the melon in half and detail the flesh into balls using a Parisian spoon.
-Step 3: Cut the cherry tomatoes in half, the diced mozzarella and the ham into strips.
-Step 4: In a salad bowl, mix the lemon juice and the olive oil. Salt and pepper. Add 6 chopped basil leaves.
-Step 5: Drain the pasta. Pass them quickly under cold water and pour them into the salad bowl. Mix. Add the melon balls, cherry tomatoes, mozzarella, ham and olives.
-Step 6: Sprinkle with remaining basil, and Serve cold, but not to much.

Salad white cabbage and apple

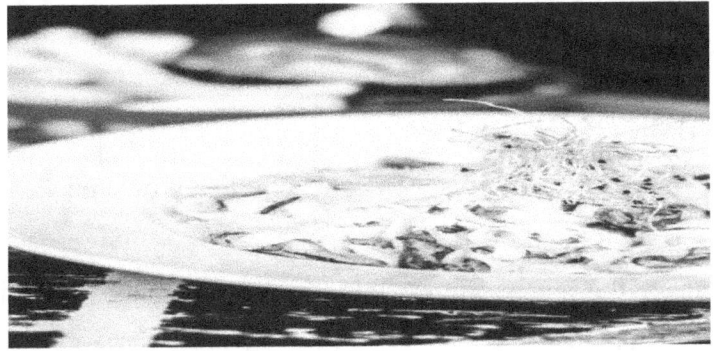

Ingredients:

-2 Apples 1 green and a granny

-2 Carrots

-4/1 White cabbage

-150g Smoked bacon

-Tablespoon of vinegar

-Small pot of mayonnaise

-Hard boiled eggs

-drops of Tabasco

-10 Cl of fresh cream

-Curry Spoon

-Pepper / Salt

Method:

Step 1:   Slice the cabbage into strips.

Step 2 cut the apples   into   small cubes without removing the skin.

Step 3:   Grated carrots.

Step 4: cut the eggs into small cubes.

Step 5: Brown the bacon.

Step 6: Put cabbage, carrots, apples, bacon in a bowl and stir.

Step 7: Sprinkle with the eggs.

Step 8: Make the sauce with mayonnaise, vinegar, Tabasco curry, salt and pepper.

 Finally add the cream and pour over the salad about 15 minutes before serving.

Cold salad with potatoes

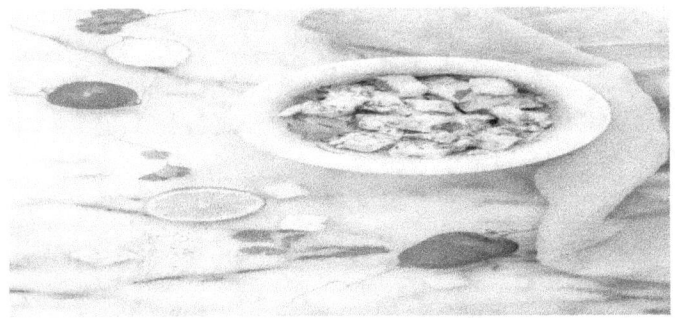

Ingredients:

500g Potatoes

2 Spoon with mayonnaise soup

2 Onions

10 Pickles or 5 big

2 Tablespoons of vinegar

Good pinch of salt

Method:

Step 1: Boil the potatoes until cooked, but not as much as for a mashed potato.
Step 2: Peel and cut the potatoes. Cut onions and pickles into small pieces.
Step 3: Mix all the ingredients.
Step 4: Put in the refrigerator.

Greek salad

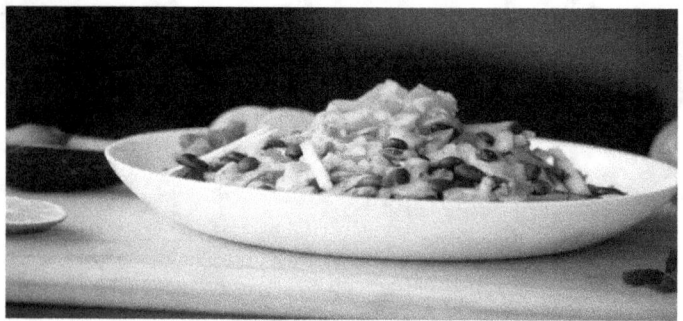

Ingredients:

-2 Tomatoes
-2/1 Cucumber diced
-Green and 1 red pepper, seeded and cut into thin slices
-150g Feta in cubes
-Onion cut into thin slices
-Lemon zest
-1 Teaspoon dried oregano
-50g Black olives facultative
-Salt / pepper

Method:

Step 1: Cut the tomatoes into small cubes and put them in a salad bowl.
Step 2: Add the cucumber, green pepper and olives.
Step 3: Mix with half of the onion and the diced feta cheese.
Step 4: Arrange remaining onion and feta on the top of the salad.
Step 5: Add zest and lemon juice, season with oil and oregano, salt pepper.
Step 6: Mix gently and serve, Delicious food.

Multicolored summer fruit salad

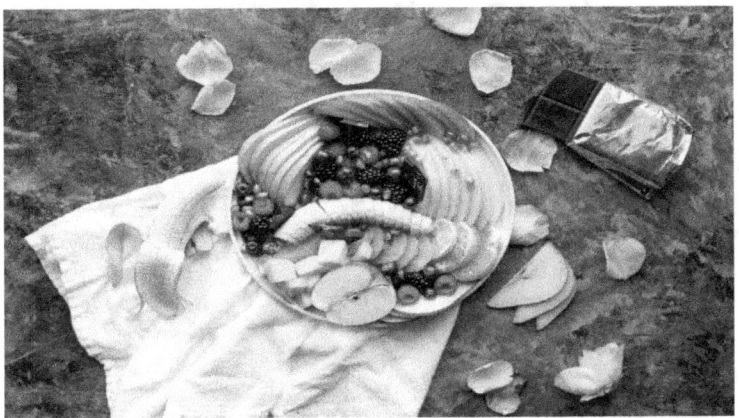

Ingredients:

-1 Fresh pineapple
-250g Strawberries gariguettes
-200g Of currants
-2 Bananas
-1 Big apple
-2 Pears
-2 White peaches
-2 Yellow nectarines
-2 Kiwis
-1/4 Watermelon
-1/2 Melon
-2 Limes

Method:

1: Cut the pineapple into very small pieces, add the strawberries, the lemon banana slices, the lemon-flavored apple and pear cubes, the peach and nectarine cubes, the kiwi slices, the watermelon bubbles and melon.
2: Sprinkle with creams and decorate with fresh mint.

Soft Fish Soup

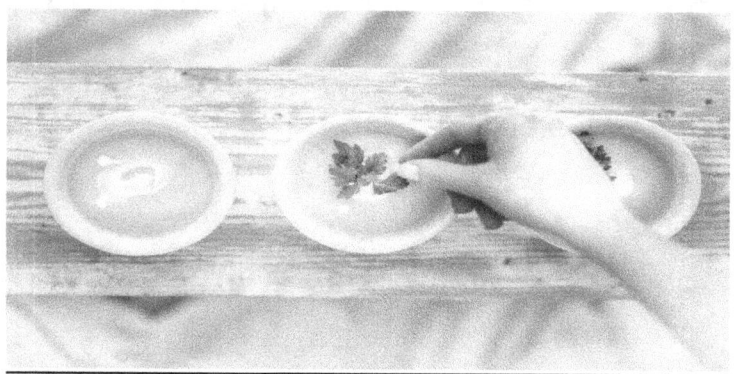

Ingredients:

-1/2 kg fish is recommended to be a mix of different types

-1 Large onion

-2 Fresh tomatoes

-5 Cloves of garlic, Salt, Black pepper, Cumin, Metalus, and two eaves of rand.

-A little table oil

Method:

- Put the fish after cleaning it in a vase with a little salt and let it boil on low heat for about 10 minutes, and on the one hand put onions, oil, salt, garlic, metal, pepper, cumin, rand and tomatoes in a saucepan to be fried, Then boil it with thyme and put it in the pot, add a little hot water to it, and mix for 10 minutes. Then stir the mixture with a mixing machine.

Mexican steak

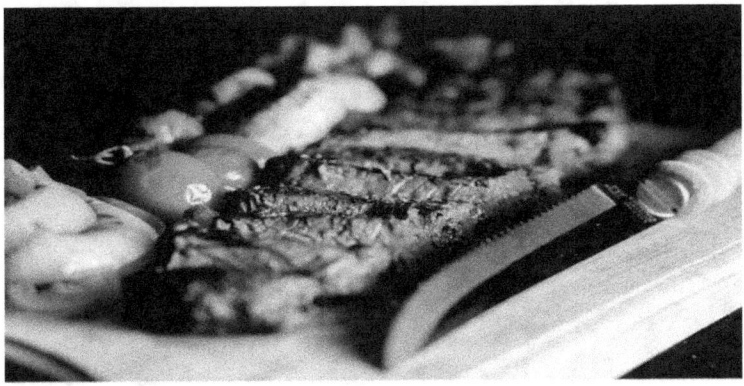

Ingredients:

4 Thick slices of beef steak

2 Medium-sized onions (small slices)

2 Chili pepper (cut into small pieces)

4 Pieces of colored peppers (cut into circles)

2 Tomatoes (finely chopped)

1 Small hanging from barbeque

2 Zucchini fruit (two circles shaped)

1/4 Cup of lemon juice

1/4 Cup olive oil

1/2 Teaspoon black pepper 4 cloves garlic mashed

Method:

First, mix the previous ingredients well except for the zucchini.
Sauce the slices well with the previous mixture and leave them in the fridge for 2 to 3 hours.
 Place the meat, sausage and vegetables on the charcoal for at least 15 minutes.
Place the steak in the serving dish and add to it Vegetables.

Eggplant Kebab

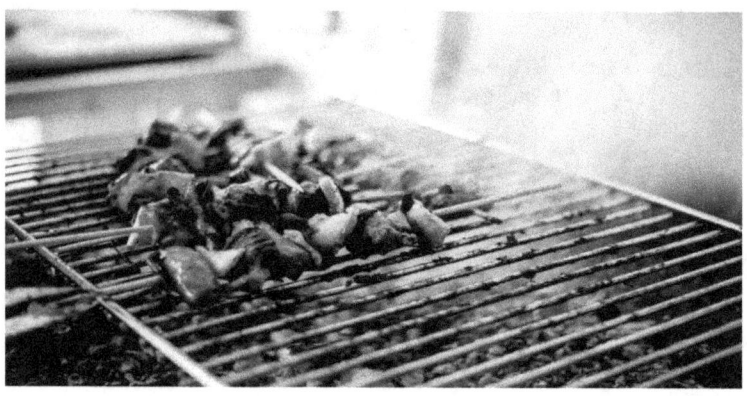

Ingredients:

-1/2 kg Minced meat
-1 Onion powder
-2 Garlic cloves and black pepper
-1/2 Teaspoon hot red pepper
-4 Eggplant slice circles
-1 Tbsp olive oil
-A Pinch of salt

Method:

Mix all the kebabs in a bowl to become homogenous.
Take pieces of meat and shape into medium sized balls.
Take it to the refrigerator.
To prepare the eggplant: sprinkle the salt on the slides and leave it aside for 30 minutes.
Apply it with a dry cloth to get rid of the juices.
Put it in a bowl with olive oil and black pepper with black pepper.
Shape the meatballs alternately with the eggplant and then saute it on the charcoal until cooked.

Indian vegetable soup with chickpeas

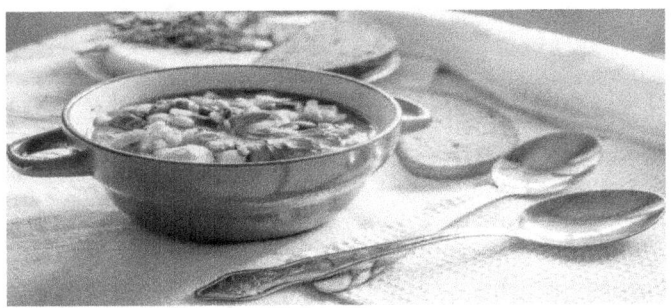

Ingredients:

-Tablespoon vegetable oil.
-Large grain of chopped onion.
-Teaspoon grated ginger.
-1/2 Teaspoon of mashed garlic.
-Spoon of Bharat Gramsala.
-850ml of chicken stock.
-Carrots cut into small squares.
-Pack of canned hummus, washed and drained from water.
-100g Green beans or beans, minced.

Method:

Heat the oil in a saucepan over medium heat.
Add onions, garlic and ginger to the saucepan and the ingredients for 2 minutes.
 Add the bharat gharamasala and let it taste fresh for about 1 minute and then pour the chicken broth and carrots.
Cook for 10 minutes after simmering on low heat.
Add the chickpeas to the soup, using the electric grinder.
Mix the soup until you get the creamy soup.
Add the beans.
 Add the soup for another three minutes, and then remove the soup from the fire.

<u>Chapter 7</u>

Supplementary advice on diet, sleep and its relationship to low weight.

Get enough sleep every day

Take care to get enough sleep every day. The body repairs itself during sleep, regulates stress, hunger hormones, cortisol, and glycine, the higher the levels of the hormone petiole and the glycine, the more people eat. It is always advisable to set up a sleeping table, where specific sleep times are set.

Organizing meals

It is important to eat at regular times during the day. This helps to burn calories faster. This method helps to reduce the intake of snacks between meals that contain high levels of fat and sugars, and be careful not to skip breakfast, It is one of the most important meals, because skipping is not getting the basic nutrients, and increasing the need to eat more snacks throughout the day.

Conclusion

Today we completed this book, hope you liked it, and helped us achieve your goal of weight loss, thank you so much for your trust in this book.

The End

www.ingramcontent.com/pod-product-compliance
Lightning Source LLC
Chambersburg PA
CBHW070306290526
45791CB00003B/1094